The Dash Diet Cookbook for Beginners 2021

Try New Mouthwatering Recipes to Boost Your Immune System, Lower Pressure and Prevent Diabetes

Pamela Holland

Disclaimer Notice:

Please note the information contained within this document is for educational and entertainment purposes only. All effort has been executed to present accurate, up to date, and reliable, complete information. No warranties of any kind are declared or implied. Readers acknowledge that the author is not engaging in the rendering of legal, financial, medical or professional advice. The content within this book has been derived from various sources. Please consult a licensed professional before attempting any techniques outlined in this book.

By reading this document, the reader agrees that under no circumstances is the author responsible for any losses, direct or indirect, which are incurred as a result of the use of information contained within this document, including, but not limited to, errors, omissions, or inaccuracies.

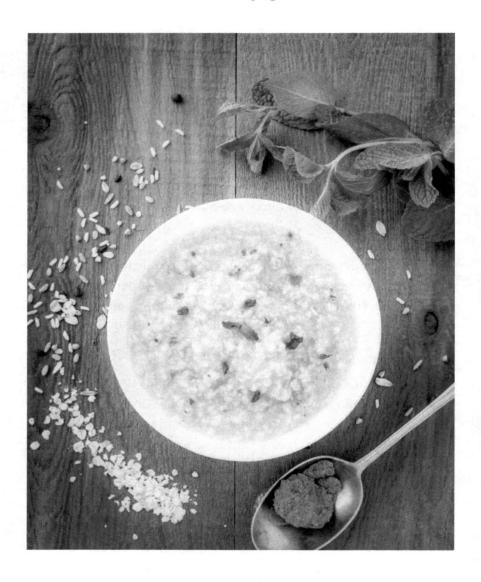

Table of Contents

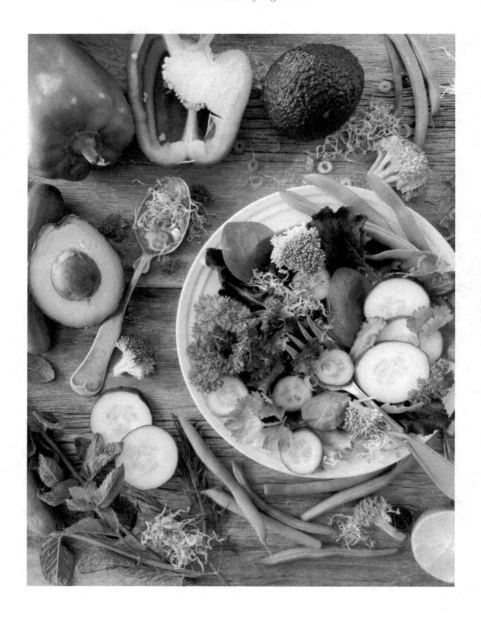

INTRODUCTION

How DASH diet came about?

The experts of the Institute of Health Planning Studies in Baltimore, Maryland suggested that the government should have a diet which would decrease the risk of heart diseases, lower blood pressure and control the sodium levels of food. Though the main focus of this diet was to stop the progression of hypertension and heart disease, the diet was also recommended for people who are obese, overweight, multiply diabetic and elderly. The list of food items which were good for lowering blood pressure was published in early 1993. The name 'DASH diet' was officially used in the summer of 1993, for the first time. The outcome of this diet was given great importance since it was known to work.

DASH diet is a healthy eating plan which is recommended for people over the age of fifty and who are obese and have high blood pressure. The diet includes fruits and vegetables in abundance and there are reduced fatty, sodium and cholesterol. The diet aims to give your body more energy. It aims to stop your intake of sodium and to include the food items that are good in lowering blood pressure.This diet is basically based on the recommendations of the National Heart, Lung and Blood Institute. When the Department of Health and Human Services found that there was a need for an alternative diet which would control the sodium levels of food and would help in lowering the risk of disease, they took over the initiative to conduct research. The Institute of Health Planning Studies carried out a lot of research regarding a diet which would be healthy and would lower blood pressure. The recommendations of this institute were published in 1993. The recommendation was for people who are over the age of fifty, overweight, obese and who had high blood pressure. The diet was originally introduced as the 'Dietary Approaches to Stop Hypertension' (DASH) diet. It was a well-balanced diet which had the recommended amount of food groups. The principles of the DASH diet were also followed by the government.The main objective of this diet was to lower the risk of developing a stroke, hypertension and heart disease. The nutrients in the diet were also well balanced to keep you healthy.

DASH DIET OVERVIEW

Benefits Of Dash Diet

A few preliminaries have been completed to help recognize and evaluate the benefits of the DASH diet. These include:

- Reduction in blood pressure - in only two weeks of following the DASH diet, the blood pressure frequently drops a couple of focuses, and whenever persevered in, this could bring about the systolic blood pressure descending by eight to fourteen focuses.

- The DASH diet additionally improves bone quality and forestalls osteoporosis due to expanded calcium consumption from dairy items and verdant green vegetables.

- A high admission of new or solidified fruits and vegetables is related to a lower danger of disease in the long haul.

- The metabolic issues, for example, cardiovascular ailment and diabetes, just as cerebrovascular illness, are diminished by the reasonable food admission with the DASH diet, prompting lowered fat utilization and expanded substitution of complex starches for straightforward sugars. This prompts an abatement in the aggregate and LDL cholesterol in the blood, just as a reduction in blood pressure.

- A lowered danger of gout by lessening corrosive uric levels in subjects with hyperuricemia is an extra advantage of the DASH diet.

Subsequently, the DASH diet is not an accident or hardship diet yet one that allows for complete nutrition and long haul foundation of healthy eating. To diminish sodium utilization, even more, a low sodium variant of the DASH diet is likewise accessible. This decreases sodium to 1500 mg daily from the standard 2300 mg/day, which itself is a significant enhancement for the normal American diet.

Food to Eat and To Avoid

What to Eat

This is one of the meals that have a history of being eaten in the wrong way. Most people don't know the proper meal plan for breakfast because they are not used to eat. Well, do not worry; I got your back on that. Below are some right choices preferred for breakfast in the morning?

Eggs - according to most research, eggs are one of the most preferred meals in the morning and are used to help reduce blood sugar in the body especially the egg yolk.

Greek yogurt - yogurt is rich in proteins and provides energy in the body. Yogurt is mostly preferred because they keep the stomach full for long before they feel empty again.

Coffee - those who do or spent a lot of times in the office prefer coffee to tea mainly because coffee is well known to ensure that the body remains alert and the mood is often jovial.

Nuts - nuts are not only sweet and tasty in nature, but they are also very important when it comes to monitoring the body weight to ensure you don't get fat to obesity.

What to have for lunch

Some say breakfast is more important than lunch, some argue that the vice versa is true. Well, personally, don't let anyone fool you otherwise. Lunch is a very important part of the meal and is there mainly to help you get through the afternoon with a full stomach. Lunch is more effective especially when it is taken in the right way and in the right proportion. Below are some of the best options to consider for your lunchtime hour.

- Vegetables

- Sandwich
- Chicken salad
- Chips
- Black beans
- Potatoes

Lunch is important in various ways. For instance, lunch is important because it helps to increase the blood sugar during the day which results in concentration and alertness for the rest of the afternoon. Skipping lunch for those who take it likely should know that is very wrong and comes with severe consequences especially when you are working or a student. This is because when you skip lunch, chances of distractions and lots of attention in classes are very high which leads to poor performance at the end of the day.

What to have for supper

Supper is one of the hectic times in the meal plan and most people find it hard to stick to, especially the bachelors living alone. This is the people who leave for work early and return to the house late at night with tired bodies and mind. At this point, the mind is mostly tired and it just wants you to go to the shower, take a warm clean bath, and go to sleep till the next day. That occurs in a lot of times to most workers especially the low wage workers who are underpaid and work the most hours. Below are some simple foods you can prepare for your supper that get cooked and are ready within a short time.

- Spaghetti
- Beef stew
- Tuna and avocado
- Chicken bake
- Scrambled eggs
- Broccoli

Those are some of the quickest foods to prepare for your supper within a short time before going to bed or if not in a hurry, you can try brown rice, fried meat, or fish.

Some foods are taken based on certain situations and many of this time there is never otherwise of any alternative. It might be a prison form of situation, where you have to eat what other people are eating and there is no other option of selection, or it might be a pregnancy situation where a mother has to eat right in order to deliver a healthy baby when due.

Having known what to eat and when to eat and why to eat, we will then focus on the don'ts of what not to eat and the worst foods never to try in your menu as a concluding part.

What Not to Eat

Microwave foods

The microwave is good for most people because they are fast to cook and save a lot of time to people especially those that prefer preparing quick foods. Well, that is good. It really helps a lot, but at the same time, the microwave is known to come with severe issues too. Like for instance, it may lead to diabetes or the fact that the food prepared is never evenly cooked.

Hot dogs

It is true that they are very sweet and tasty and most people prefer buying them during sports activities or after running in the street. Hot dogs are junk foods and are rich in fats that lead to overweight if proper actions are not taken. The major danger that comes with it is the presence of sodium in them which is not needed in the body at all.

Doughnuts

Doughnuts are the other sweet type of cakes that are loved by a lot of people because of their tasty allure. The sad truth is that these doughnuts are prepared by the GMO's which often leads to cancer when taken in excess and can even cause fast death from clogging the arteries.

Pizza

What is the first thing that comes to mind when you think of pizza? I don't know about you, but my first is that it is yummy. Pizza is the top in the list of the world eaten junk food with the most deliveries in a day. Most people love to order pizza during house parties or when left alone in the house by the parents or when there is no food in the house to eat and you are desperate for food in the stomach. Pizza is mixed with a lot of things that are rich in calories and that is the major reason why you should stop eating pizza from today.

Why Dash Diet Works?

The food plan mainly focuses on vegetables, fruits, low-fat/non-Fat dairy and whole grains. The eating plan also includes the consumption of high fiber foods, medium to low amounts of fat, low red meat, and less sugar. An additional benefit of this diet is that it is rich in different vitamins and minerals that are important in achieving a healthy body.

Another good thing about this diet plan is that it lowers your Sodium intake in your diet (daily consumption for Sodium is only 2,300 mg on the dash diet) that will help regulate blood pressure levels. That's because studies show that eating food with high sodium content could lead to a spike in blood pressure.

The diet plan has claimed to lower the blood pressure in just two weeks and has been recommended by Centers for Disease Control, American Heart Association, The National Heart, Lung and Blood Institute, the Mayo Clinic, US Government guidelines for the treatment of hypertension and a lot more.

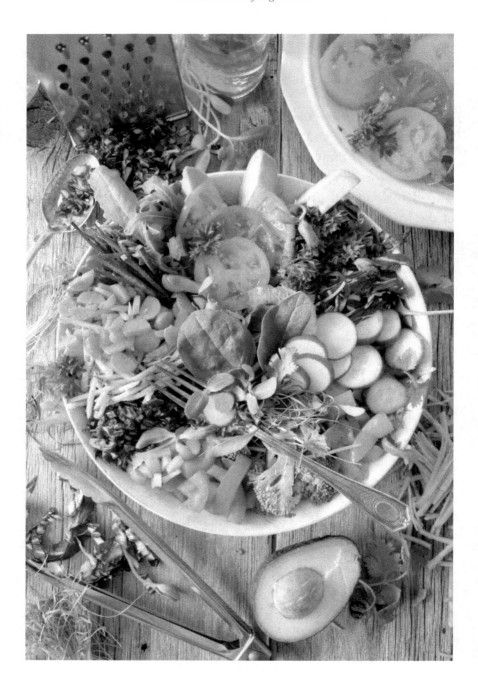

THE IMPORTANCE OF EXERCISE DURING DIET

Exercise is good for human health in many ways, regardless of what you choose to do. My goal in this section is not only to gently introduce you to the numerous health benefits that regular physical activity can offer but also to remind you that your 28-day plan will include a diverse, varied exercise routine that I hope provides options that everyone can get something out of.

Although the DASH diet focuses on food choices, there is no denying that regular and varied exercise represents an important component of a healthy lifestyle and one that can confer additional benefits. For those of you who are starting from square one, you should know that any exercise is better than none and that there is absolutely nothing wrong with starting slowly and easing into a more rigorous routine. With that being said, the CDC identifies moderate intensity aerobic activity that totals 120 to 150 minutes weekly, in combination with two additional weekly days of muscular resistance training, as an ideal combination to confer numerous health benefits to adults. Per the CDC, these benefits include the following:

Better weight management: When combined with dietary modification, regular physical activity plays a role in supporting or enhancing weight-management efforts. Regular exercise is a great way to expend calories on top of any dietary changes you will be making on this program.

Reduced risk for cardiovascular disease: A reduction in blood pressure is a well-recognized benefit of regular physical activity, which ultimately contributes to a reduced risk of cardiovascular disease.

Reduced risk of type 2 diabetes: Regular physical activity is known to improve blood glucose control and insulin sensitivity.

Improved mood: Regular physical activity is associated with improvements in mood and reductions in anxiety owing to the manner in which exercise positively influences the biochemistry of the human brain by releasing hormones and affecting neurotransmitters.

A longer life span: Those who exercise regularly tend to enjoy a lower risk of chronic disease and a longer life span.

As you will see in the 28-day plan, your recommended exercise totals will be met by exercising four out of the seven days a week. The exercise days will be broken up as follows: All four of the active days will include aerobic exercise for 30 minutes. As a beginner, I encourage you to start slowly and build up to the four days. Two of the four active days will also include strength training. The bottom line is that you don't have to exercise for hours each day to enjoy the health benefits of physical activity. Our goal with this plan is to make the health benefits of exercise as accessible and attainable as possible for those who are ready and willing to give it a try. Before we get to the good stuff, though, there is still a lot of wisdom to be shared about getting the most out of your workouts.

GETTING THE MOST OUT OF YOUR WORKOUTS

Just as with healthy eating strategies, there are certainly important things to keep in mind about physical activity that will help support your long-term success. Let's take a look at a few important considerations that will help you get the most out of your workouts:

Rest days: Even though we haven't even started, I'm going to preach the importance of good rest. Don't forget that you are taking part in this journey to improve your health for the long term, not to burn yourself out in 28 days. Although some of you with more experience with exercise may feel confident going above and beyond, my best advice for the majority of those reading is to listen to your body and take days off to minimize risk of injury and burnout.

Stretching: Stretching is a great way to prevent injury and keep you pain-free both during workouts and in daily life. Whether it's a deliberate activity after a workout or through additional means such as yoga, stretching is beneficial in many ways.

Enjoyment: There is no right or wrong style of exercise. You are being provided a diverse plan that emphasizes a variety of different cardiovascular and resistance training exercises. If there are certain activities within these groups that you don't enjoy, it's okay not to do them. Your ability to stick with regular physical activity in the long term will depend on finding a style of exercise that you enjoy.

Your limits: Physical activity is good for you, and it should be fun, too. It's up to you to keep it that way. While it is important to challenge yourself, don't risk injury by taking things too far too fast.

Your progress: Although this is not an absolute requirement, some of you reading may find joy and fulfillment through tracking your exercise progress and striving toward a longer duration, more repetitions, and so on. If you are the type who enjoys a competitive edge, it may be fun to find a buddy to exercise and progress with.

Warm-ups: Last but certainly not least, your exercise routine will benefit greatly from a proper warm-up routine, which includes starting slowly or doing exercises similar to the ones included in your workout, but at a lower intensity.

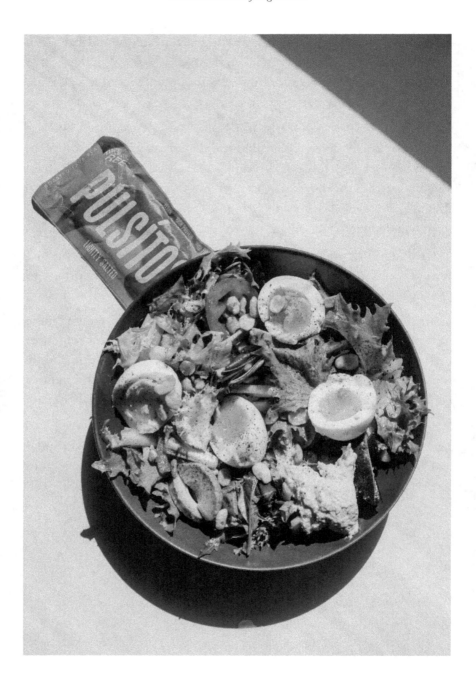

THE 28-DAY PROGRAM

DAY	BREAKFAST	LUNCH	DINNER	SNACKS
1	Sweet Potatoes with Coconut Flakes	Stuffed Mushrooms Caps	Decent Beef and Onion Stew	Coconut Peppers Dip
2	Flaxseed & Banana Smoothie	Beef with Pea Pods	Clean Parsley and Chicken Breast	Lentils Dip
3	Fruity Tofu Smoothie	Whole-Grain Rotini with Ground Pork	Zucchini Beef Sauté with Coriander Greens	Coconut Cranberry Crackers
4	French toast with Applesauce	Roasted Pork Loin with Herbs	Hearty Lemon and Pepper Chicken	Chili Walnuts
5	Banana-Peanut Butter 'n Greens Smoothie	Garlic Lime Pork Chops	Walnuts and Asparagus Delight	Coconut Cranberry Crackers
6	Baking Powder Biscuits	Lamb Curry with Tomatoes and Spinach	Healthy Carrot Chips	Almond Bars
7	Oatmeal	Pomegranate-	Amazing	Almond

	Banana Pancakes with Walnuts	Marinated Leg of Lamb	Grilled Chicken and Blueberry Salad	Bowls
8	Creamy Oats, Greens & Blueberry Smoothie	Shrimp Lunch Rolls	Elegant Pumpkin Chili Dish	Paprika Potato Chips
9	Banana & Cinnamon Oatmeal	Turkey Sandwich with Mozzarella	Zucchini Zoodles with Chicken and Basil	Coconut Kale Spread
10	Bagels Made Healthy	Vegetable Tacos	Tasty Roasted Broccoli	Cumin Beets Chips
11	Cereal with Cranberry-Orange Twist	Sausage with Potatoes	The Almond Breaded Chicken Goodness	Dill Zucchini Spread
12	No Cook Overnight Oats	Crunchy Fried Chicken	South-Western Pork Chops	Seeds Bowls
13	Avocado Cup with Egg	Roasted Salmon with Chives and Tarragon	Chicken Salsa	Tahini Pumpkin Dip

14	Mediterranean Toast	Stuffed Mushrooms Caps	Brown Butter Duck Breast	Cheesy Spinach Dip
15	Instant Banana Oatmeal	Beef with Pea Pods	Decent Beef and Onion Stew	Coconut Peppers Dip
16	Flaxseed & Banana Smoothie	Whole-Grain Rotini with Ground Pork	Clean Parsley and Chicken Breast	Lentils Dip
17	Fruity Tofu Smoothie	Roasted Pork Loin with Herbs	Zucchini Beef Sauté with Coriander Greens	Coconut Cranberry Crackers
18	French toast with Applesauce	Garlic Lime Pork Chops	Hearty Lemon and Pepper Chicken	Chili Walnuts
19	Banana-Peanut Butter 'n Greens Smoothie	Lamb Curry with Tomatoes and Spinach	Walnuts and Asparagus Delight	Coconut Cranberry Crackers
20	Baking Powder Biscuits	Pomegranate-Marinated Leg of Lamb	Healthy Carrot Chips	Almond Bars
21	Oatmeal	Shrimp	Amazing	Almond

	Banana Pancakes with Walnuts	Lunch Rolls	Grilled Chicken and Blueberry Salad	Bowls
22	Creamy Oats, Greens & Blueberry Smoothie	Turkey Sandwich with Mozzarella	Elegant Pumpkin Chili Dish	Paprika Potato Chips
23	Banana & Cinnamon Oatmeal	Vegetable Tacos	Zucchini Zoodles with Chicken and Basil	Coconut Kale Spread
24	Bagels Made Healthy	Sausage with Potatoes	Tasty Roasted Broccoli	Cumin Beets Chips
25	Cereal with Cranberry-Orange Twist	Crunchy Fried Chicken	The Almond Breaded Chicken Goodness	Dill Zucchini Spread
26	No Cook Overnight Oats	Roasted Salmon with Chives and Tarragon	South-Western Pork Chops	Seeds Bowls
27	Avocado Cup with Egg	Stuffed Mushrooms Caps	Chicken Salsa	Tahini Pumpkin Dip

Shopping List

Vegetables

- Acorn Squash

- Artichokes

- Asparagus

- Beets

- Bell peppers, any color

- Broccoli

- Brussels sprouts

- Butternut squash

- Cabbage

- Carrots

- Cauliflower

- Celery

- Collard greens

- Cucumbers

- Eggplant

- Green beans

- Jicama

- Kale

- Mushrooms

- Leeks

- Lettuce

- Onions, any color

- Parsnips
- Peas
- Potatoes (limit for weight loss)
- Pumpkin
- Radishes
- Rutabaga
- Spaghetti squash
- Spinach
- Sweet potatoes (limit for weight loss)
- Swiss chard
- Summer squash
- Tomatoes
- Turnips
- Turnip Greens
- Zucchini

Fruits

- Apples
- Apricots
- Bananas
- Blackberries
- Blueberries
- Cantaloupe
- Cherries
- Dates

- Figs
- Grapefruit
- Grapes
- Honeydew Melon
- Kiwi fruit
- Lemon
- Lime
- Mango
- Nectarines
- Oranges
- Papaya
- Peaches
- Pears
- Pineapple
- Plums
- Prunes
- Raisins
- Raspberries
- Strawberries
- Tangerines
- Watermelon

Dairy (always choose low fat or fat free options when available)

- Buttermilk
- Cottage cheese

- Fresh cheeses such as feta, fresh mozzarella, queso, etc.
- Hard cheeses such as cheddar, Colby, Monterey Jack, Asiago, Parmesan, etc.
- Kefir
- Margarine, trans fat free varieties
- Milk
- Ricotta cheese
- Soft cheeses, such as blue, gorgonzola, Brie, etc.
- Sour cream
- Yogurt

Lean Meat, Poultry, and Seafood

- Beef, ground (lean)
- Beef roast
- Beef steak (lean)
- Chicken, skinless, preferably light meat pieces
- Chicken, ground
- Deli meat, low sodium
- Eggs
- Fresh fish
- Pork tenderloin
- Shrimp and other seafood
- Tempeh
- Tofu
- Turkey, skinless, preferably light meat pieces

- Turkey, ground

Nuts, Seeds, and Legumes

- Almonds

- Cashews

- Dry beans

- Hazelnuts

- Nut butters

- Peanuts

- Pecans

- Pistachios

- Pumpkin seeds

- Soy nuts

- Sunflower seeds

- Walnuts

Condiments

   Chili garlic sauce

- Dijon mustard

- Hot sauce

- Hummus

- Jams or Jellies, fruit only or sugar free

- Marinara sauce, low sodium

- Mayonnaise, low fat

- Oils, such as olive or canola

- Salsa, fresh

- Salad dressing, low fat
- Soft or liquid margarine trans-fat free

Suggested Seasonings

- Cayenne pepper
- Chili powder
- Chives
- Cilantro
- Cinnamon
- Cloves
- Coriander
- Crushed red pepper flakes
- Cumin
- Curry powder
- Dill
- Garlic powder
- Ginger
- Nutmeg
- Oregano
- Paprika
- Parsley
- Pepper:
- Rosemary
- Sage
- Tarragon

BREAKFAST

1. **Bagels Made Healthy**

Preparation time: 5 minutes

Cooking time: 40 minutes

Servings: 8

Ingredients:

- 1 ½ c. warm water

- 1 ¼ c. bread flour

- 2 tbsps. Honey

- 2 c. whole wheat flour

- 2 tsps. Yeast

- 1 ½ tbsps. Olive oil

- 1 tbsp. vinegar

Directions:

1. In a bread machine, mix all ingredients, and then process on dough cycle.

2. Once done, create 8 pieces shaped like a flattened ball.

3. Make a hole in the center of each ball using your thumb then create a donut shape.

4. In a greased baking sheet, place donut-shaped dough then cover and let it rise about ½ hour.

5. Prepare about 2 inches of water to boil in a large pan.

6. In boiling water, drop one at a time the bagels and boil for 1 minute, then turn them once.

7. Remove them and return to baking sheet and bake at 350oF for about 20 to 25 minutes until golden brown.

Nutrition: Calories: 228.1, Fat: 3.7 g Carbs: 41.8 g Protein: 6.9 g Sugars: 0 g Sodium: 15%

2. **<u>Cereal with Cranberry-Orange Twist</u>**

Preparation time: 5 minutes

Cooking time: 0 minutes

Servings: 1

Ingredients:

- ½ c. water

- ½ c. orange juice

- 1/3 c. oat bran

- ¼ c. dried cranberries

- Sugar

- Milk

Directions:

1. In a bowl, combine all ingredients.

2. For about 2 minutes, microwave the bowl then serve with sugar and milk.

3. Enjoy!

Nutrition: Calories: 220.4, Fat: 2.4 g Carbs: 43.5 g Protein: 6.2 g Sugars: 8 g Sodium: 1%

3. **No Cook Overnight Oats**

Preparation time: 5 minutes

Cooking time: 0 minutes

Servings: 1

Ingredients:

- 1 ½ c. low Fat milk

- 5 whole almond pieces

- 1 tsp. chia seeds

- 2 tbsps. Oats

- 1 tsp. sunflower seeds

- 1 tbsp. Craisins

Directions:

1. In a jar or mason bottle with cap, mix all ingredients.

2. Refrigerate overnight.

3. Enjoy for breakfast. Will keep in the fridge for up to 3 days.

Nutrition: Calories: 271, Fat: 9.8 g Carbs: 35.4 g Protein: 16.7 g Sugars: 9 Sodium: 103%

LUNCH RECIPES

4. **Vegetable Tacos**

Preparation Time: 30 minutes

Cooking Time: 30 minutes

Servings: 4

Ingredients:

- 1 Tablespoon Olive Oil

- 1 Cup Red Onion, Chopped

- 1 Cup Yellow Summer Squash, Diced

- 1 Cup Green Zucchini, Diced

- 3 Cloves Garlic, Minced

- 4 Tomatoes, Seeded& Chopped

- 1 Jalapeno Chili, Seeded & Chopped

- 1 Cup Corn Kernels, Fresh

- 1 Cup Pinto Beans, Canned, Rinsed & Drained

- ½ Cup Cilantro, Fresh & Chopped

- 8 Corn Tortillas

- ½ Cup Smoke Flavored Salsa

Directions:

1. Get out a saucepan and add in your olive oil over medium heat, and stir in your onion. Cook until softened.

2. Add in your squash and zucchini, cooking for an additional five minutes.

3. Stir in your garlic, beans, tomatoes, jalapeño and corn. Cook for an additional five minutes before stirring in your cilantro and removing the pan from heat.

4. Warm each tortilla, in a nonstick skillet for twenty seconds per side.

5. Place the tortillas on a serving plate, spooning the vegetable mixture into each. Top with salsa, and roll to serve.

Nutrition: Calories: 310 Protein: 10 g Fat: 6 g Carbs: 54 g Sodium: 97 mg Cholesterol: 20 mg

5. <u>**Sausage with Potatoes**</u>

Preparation time: 10 minutes

Cooking time: 22 minutes

Servings: 6

Ingredients:

- ½ pound smoked sausage, cooked and chopped

- 3 tablespoons olive oil

- 1 and ¾ pounds red potatoes, cubed

- 2 yellow onions, chopped

- 1 teaspoon thyme, dried

- 2 teaspoons cumin, ground

- A pinch of black pepper

Directions:

1. Heat up a pan with the oil over medium-high heat, add potatoes and onions, stir and cook for 12 minutes.

2. Add sausage, thyme, cumin and black pepper, stir, cook for 10 minutes more, divide between plates and serve for lunch.

3. Enjoy!

Nutrition: Calories 199, Fat 2, Fiber 4, Carbs 14, Protein 8 Sodium 24%

6. <u>**Crunchy Fried Chicken**</u>

Preparation Time: 50 minutes

Cooking Time: 45 minutes

Servings: 4

Ingredients:

- One-fourth tsp. salt

- One/eight tsp. dry mustard seasoning

- One-half tsp. cayenne pepper

- Two oz. cornmeal

- One-half tsp. paprika seasoning

- Two oz. cornflakes, crumbled

- Four chicken breasts, boneless and skinless

- Two tbsp. whole wheat flour

- Olive oil cooking spray

- Two oz. buttermilk, low-fat

- One tsp. garlic powder

Directions:

1. Set the stove to heat at 375° Fahrenheit. Apply a coat of olive oil spray over a 9-inch glass baking dish.

2. Empty the buttermilk into a glass dish.

3. In an additional dish, blend the cornflakes, cornmeal, and flour with a whisk to integrate.

4. Season with the mustard, cayenne pepper, paprika, garlic powder, and salt and combine fully.

5. Immerse one chicken breast first in the buttermilk and then into the cornflakes to completely cover the meat. Make sure the chicken is not dripping by removing any excess batter.

6. Transfer the coated chicken to the prepped baking dish.

7. Repeat steps 5 and 6 for the remaining chicken.

8. Apply the olive oil spray to the chicken and heat in the stove for half an hour.

9. Remove and enjoy immediately while hot.

Nutrition: Sodium: 481 mg Protein: 45 g Fat: 7 g Sugar: 1 g Calories: 540

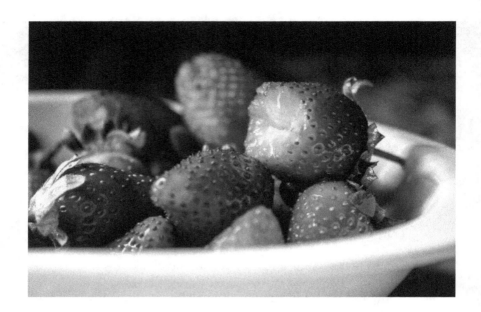

DINNER RECIPES

7. <u>Zucchini Zoodles with Chicken and Basil</u>

Preparation Time: 10 minutes

Cooking Time: 10 minutes

Servings: 2

Ingredients:

- 2 chicken fillets, cubed
- 2 tablespoons ghee
- 1 pound tomatoes, diced
- ½ cup basil, chopped
- ¼ cup coconut almond milk
- 1 garlic clove, peeled, minced
- 1 zucchini, shredded

Directions:

1. Sauté cubed chicken in ghee until no longer pink.
2. Add tomatoes and season with sunflower seeds.
3. Simmer and reduce the liquid.
4. Prepare your zucchini Zoodles by shredding zucchini in a food processor.

5. Add basil, garlic, coconut almond milk to chicken and cook for a few minutes.

6. Add half of the zucchini Zoodles to a bowl and top with creamy tomato basil chicken.

7. Enjoy!

Nutrition: Calories: 540 Fat: 27g Carbohydrates: 13g Protein: 59g

8. **Tasty Roasted Broccoli**

Preparation Time: 5 minutes

Cooking Time: 20 minutes

Servings: 4

Ingredients:

- 4 cups broccoli florets
- 1 tablespoon olive oil
- Sunflower seeds and pepper to taste

Directions:

1. Pre-heat your oven to 400 degrees F.
2. Add broccoli in a zip bag alongside oil and shake until coated.
3. Add seasoning and shake again.
4. Spread broccoli out on baking sheet, bake for 20 minutes.
5. Let it cool and serve.

Nutrition: Calories: 62 Fat: 4g Carbohydrates: 4g Protein: 4g

9. **<u>The Almond Breaded Chicken Goodness</u>**

Preparation Time: 15 minutes

Cooking Time: 15 minutes

Servings: 3

Ingredients:

- 2 large chicken breasts, boneless and skinless

- 1/3 cup lemon juice

- 1 ½ cups seasoned almond meal

- 2 tablespoons coconut oil

- Lemon pepper, to taste

- Parsley for decoration

Directions:

1. Slice chicken breast in half.

2. Pound out each half until ¼ inch thick.

3. Take a pan and place it over medium heat, add oil and heat it up.

4. Dip each chicken breast slice into lemon juice and let it sit for 2 minutes.

5. Turnover and the let the other side sit for 2 minutes as well.

6. Transfer to almond meal and coat both sides.

7. Add coated chicken to the oil and fry for 4 minutes per side, making sure to sprinkle lemon pepper liberally.

8. Transfer to a paper lined sheet and repeat until all chicken are fried.

9. Garnish with parsley and enjoy!

Nutrition: Calories: 325 Fat: 24g Carbohydrates: 3g Protein: 16g

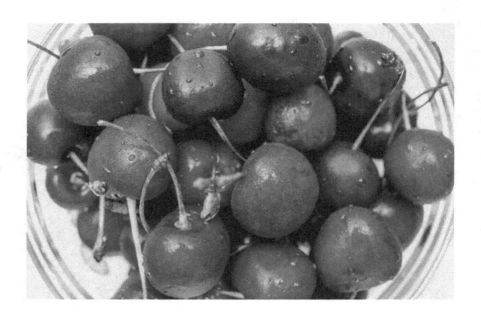

VEGETARIAN & VEGAN MAINS

10. **Portobello-Mushroom Cheeseburgers**

Preparation Time: 5 minutes

Cook Time: 10 minutes

Servings: 4

Ingredients:

- 4 Portobello mushrooms, caps removed and brushed clean

- 1 tablespoon olive oil

- ½ teaspoon freshly ground black pepper

- 1 tablespoon red wine vinegar

- 4 slices reduced-fat Swiss cheese, sliced thin

- 4 whole-wheat 100-calorie sandwich thins

- ½ avocado, sliced thin

Directions:

1. Heat a skillet or grill pan over medium-high heat. Clean the mushrooms and remove the stems. Brush each cap with olive oil and sprinkle with black pepper. Place in skillet, cap-side up and cook for about 4 minutes. Flip and cook for another 4 minutes.

2. Sprinkle with the red wine vinegar and turn over. Add the cheese and cook for 2 more minutes. For optimal melting, place a lid loosely over the pan.

3. Toast the sandwich thins. Create your burgers by topping each with sliced avocado.

4. Enjoy immediately.

Nutrition: Per Serving Total Calories: 245; Total Fat: 12g; Saturated Fat: 3g; Cholesterol: 15mg; Sodium: 266mg; Potassium: 507mg; Total Carbohydrates: 28g; Fiber: 8g; Sugars: 4g; Protein: 14g

11. <u>**Rotelle Pasta with Sun-Dried Tomato**</u>

Preparation Time: 10 minutes

Cooking Time: 20 minutes

Servings: 4

Ingredients:

- 2 tablespoons olive oil
- 4 garlic cloves, mashed
- 1/3 cup dry-packed sun-dried tomatoes, soaked in water to rehydrate, drained and chopped
- 1 3/4 cups unsalted vegetable broth
- 8 ounces uncooked whole-wheat rotelle pasta
- 1/2 cup sliced black olives (about 15 medium olives)
- 1/2 cup chopped fresh parsley
- 4 teaspoons parmesan cheese

Directions:

1. Preheat olive oil in a skillet over medium heat.
2. Sauté garlic for 30 seconds. Then add tomatoes and broth.
3. Cover the mixture and then simmer for 10 minutes.
4. Fill a pot with water and boil pasta in it for 10 minutes until al dente.
5. Drain the pasta and keep it aside.

6. Add parsley and olives to the tomato mixture and mix well.

7. Serve the plate with tomato sauce and add 1 teaspoon parmesan cheese on top.

Nutrition: Calories 335 Total Fat 4. 4 g; Saturated Fat 2. 1 g; Cholesterol 10 mg; Sodium 350 mg; Total Carbohydrates 31. 2 g; Fiber 2. 7 g; Sugar 0.6 g; Protein 7. 3 g

12. **Rice Noodles with Spring Vegetables**

Preparation Time: 5 minutes

Cooking Time: 10 minutes

Servings: 2

Ingredients:

- 1 package (8 ounces) rice noodles
- 1 tablespoon peanut oil
- 1 tablespoon sesame oil
- 1 tablespoon grated fresh ginger
- 2 garlic cloves, finely chopped
- 2 tablespoons low-sodium soy sauce
- 1 cup small broccoli florets
- 1 cup fresh bean sprouts
- 8 cherry tomatoes, halved
- 1 cup chopped fresh spinach
- 2 scallions, chopped
- Crushed red chili flakes (optional)

Directions:

1. Boil the noodles in a pot filled with water for 6 minutes until al dente and then drain it thoroughly.
2. Preheat oil in a wok and sauté garlic and ginger for 30 seconds.
3. Stir in remaining ingredients, including vegetables and noodles.
4. Toss the mixture well and then serve with crushed chili flakes on top.

Nutrition: Calories 205; Total Fat 1. 1 g; Saturated Fat 2. 8 g; Cholesterol 110 mg; Sodium 749 mg; Total Carbohydrates 12. 9 g; Fiber 0.2 g; Sugar 0.2 g; Protein 63. 5 g.

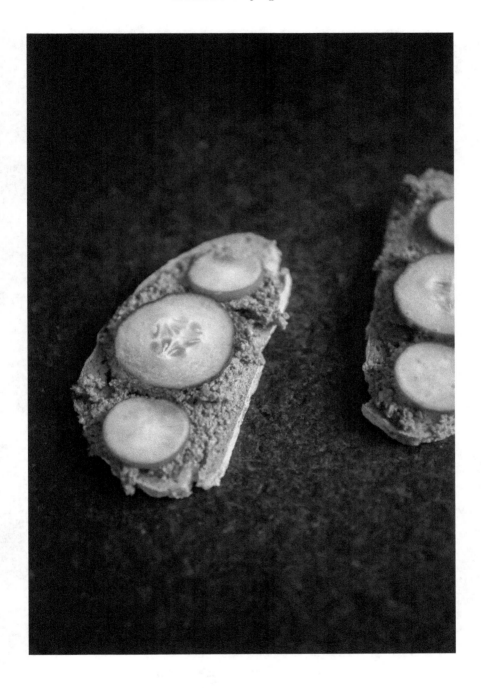

SALADS

13. **Zucchini Pesto Salad**

Preparation Time: 10 minutes

Cooking Time: 10 minutes

Servings: 4

Ingredients:

- 2 cups spiral pasta

- 2 zucchini, sliced and halved

- 4 tomatoes, cut

- 1 cup white mushrooms, cut

- 1 small red onion, chopped

- 2 tablespoons fresh basil leaves, chopped

- 2 tablespoons sunflower oil

- 1 tablespoon lemon juice

- Pepper and sunflower seeds to taste

Directions:

1. Cook the pasta according to the package instructions, drain and rinse under cold water.

2. Take a large bowl and add zucchini, tomatoes, mushrooms, onion, and pasta.

3. Mix well,

4. In a food processor, add oil, lemon juice, basil, blue cheese, black, and process well.

5. Pour the mixture over the salad and toss well.

6. Serve and enjoy!

Nutrition: Calories: 301 Fat: 25g Net Carbohydrates: 7g Protein: 10g

14.   **<u>Wholesome Potato and Tuna Salad</u>**

Preparation Time: 10 minutes

Cooking Time: 0 minute

Servings: 4

Ingredients:

- 1 pound baby potatoes, scrubbed, boiled
- 1 cup tuna chunks, drained
- 1 cup cherry tomatoes, halved
- 1 cup medium onion, thinly sliced
- 8 pitted black olives
- 2 medium hard-boiled eggs, sliced
- 1 head Romaine lettuce
- ¼ cup olive oil
- 2 tablespoons lemon juice
- 1 tablespoon Dijon mustard
- 1 teaspoon dill weed, chopped
- Pepper as needed

Directions:

1. Take a small glass bowl and mix in your olive oil, lemon juice, Dijon mustard and dill.

2. Season the mix with pepper and salt.

3. Add in the tuna, baby potatoes, cherry tomatoes, red onion, green beans, black olives and toss everything nicely.

4. Arrange your lettuce leaves on a beautiful serving dish to make the base of your salad.

5. Top them with your salad mixture and place the egg slices.

6. Drizzle with the previously prepared Salad Dressing.

7. Serve hot

Nutrition: Calories: 406 Fat: 22g Carbohydrates: 28g Protein: 26g

15. **Heart Warming Cauliflower Salad**

Preparation Time: 8 minutes

Cooking Time: 0 minute

Servings: 3

Ingredients:

- 1 head cauliflower, broken into florets
- 1 small onion, chopped
- 1/8 cup extra virgin olive oil
- ¼ cup apple cider vinegar
- ½ teaspoon of sea salt
- ½ teaspoon of black pepper
- ¼ cup dried cranberries
- ¼ cup pumpkin seeds

Directions:

1. Wash the cauliflower and break it up into small florets.

2. Transfer to a bowl. Whisk oil, vinegar, salt and pepper in another bowl. Add pumpkin seeds, cranberries to the bowl with dressing. Mix well and pour the dressing over the cauliflower. Add onions and toss. Chill and serve.

3. Enjoy!

Nutrition: Calories: 163 Fat: 11g Carbohydrates: 16g Protein: 3g

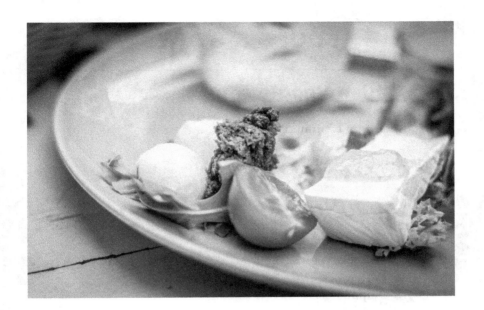

SOUPS & STEWS

16. **Italian Veggie soup**

Preparation time: 10 minutes

Cooking Time: 15 minutes

Servings: 8

Ingredients:

- 1 tablespoon olive oil

- 2 chopped carrots

- 1 cup corn

- 3 pounds peeled and chopped tomatoes

- 1 chopped celery stalk

- 1 chopped onion

- 1 chopped zucchini

- 4 minced garlic cloves

- 28 oz. Chicken stock

- 1 teaspoon Italian seasoning

- 15 oz. Kidney beans, canned, rinsed and drained

- black pepper for taste

- 2 cups baby spinach

- 2 tablespoons chopped basil

Directions:

1. Within instant pot, press sauté, heat it up and add the onion, cooking for 5 minutes.

2. Add the veggies and stir for 5 more minutes.

3. Then add spices and cook on high for 4 minutes on manual.

4. Add the spinach and beans, stirring and serving.

Nutrition: Calories: 210, Fat: 6g, Carbs: 18g, Net Carbs: 9g, Protein: 98g, Fiber: 9g

17. **Taco Soup**

Preparation time: 10 minutes

Cooking Time: 10 minutes

Servings: 4

Ingredients:

- 1 cup ground beef, cooked

- ¼ teaspoons alt

- 3 teaspoons ranch dressing mix

- 6 oz. Diced tomatoes

- 1 cup canned pinto beans

- ½ cup diced onion

- ¼ teaspoon black pepper

- 2 teaspoons taco seasoning

- 1 can of canned kernel corn

- 4 oz. Diced tomatoes with chiles

Directions: Turn on IP to sauté, and then put the beef in there, cooking till browned. Put the ingredients in there. Lock it, and then cook on high pressure for 10 minutes, then natural pressure release.

Nutrition: Calories: 200, Fat: 5g, Carbs: 12g, Net Carbs: 6g, Protein: 15g, Fiber: 6g

18. **<u>Ground Beef Soup with Tomatoes</u>**

Preparation time: 15 minutes

Cooking Time: 30 minutes

Servings: 4-6

Ingredients:

- 1 teaspoon olive oil

- 1 chopped medium onion

- 1 teaspoon dried thyme

- ½ pound fresh green beans

- 2 cans beef broth

- salt and pepper for taste

- 1 pound ground beef,

- 1 tablespoon minced garlic

- 1 teaspoon oregano

- 2 cans diced tomatoes with juice

- Parmesan for serving

Directions:

1. Turn on IP and then sauté the beef until browned, and add in the onion, thyme, garlic, and oregano, and cook for 3 minutes once beef is browned.

2. Add the tomatoes, and the beef broth, and let this all heat.

3. Trim the beans to cut into pieces about an inch long, and then add to pressure cooker.

4. Put it on soup function, and from there, use quick release for this, seasoning to taste, and serve hot with parmesan.

Nutrition: calories: 220, Fat: 6g, Carbs: 7g, Net Carbs: 4g, Protein: 15g, Fiber: 3g

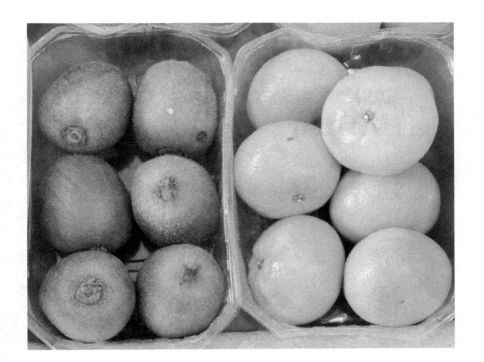

MEATLESS RECIPES

19. **Smoked Salmon Egg Scramble with Dill and Chives**

Preparation time: 5 minutes

Cooking time: 5 minutes

Servings: 2

Ingredients:

- 4 large eggs

- 1 tablespoon milk

- 1 tablespoon fresh chives, minced

- 1 tablespoon fresh dill, minced

- ¼ teaspoon kosher salt

- ⅛ teaspoon freshly ground black pepper

- 2 teaspoons extra-virgin olive oil

- 2 ounces smoked salmon, thinly sliced

Directions:

1. In a large bowl, whisk together the eggs, milk, chives, dill, salt, and pepper.

2. Heat the olive oil in a medium skillet or sauté pan over medium heat. Add the egg mixture and cook for about 3 minutes, stirring occasionally.

3. Add the salmon and cook until the eggs are set but moist, about 1 minute.

Nutrition: Calories: 325 Total fat: 26g Sodium: 455mg Total Carbohydrates: 1g Fiber: 0g Protein: 23g

20. **Deviled Eggs Guac Style**

Preparation Time: 10 minutes

Cook Time: 0 minutes

Servings: 12

Ingredients:

- 1 ripe avocado

- 1 tbsp. green onion, chopped

- 1 tbsp. Cilantro

- 1 tbsp. Lime

- 1/2 jalapeno chili pepper

- 1 tbsp. light sour cream

- 6 medium eggs, hard boiled and peeled

Directions:

1. In a medium bowl, mash avocado. Mix in green onion, cilantro, lime, pepper, and sour cream. Mix well. Slice hard boiled eggs in half lengthwise. Scoop out yolk and place in bowl of avocados. Mix well.

2. Scoop out avocado yolk mixture and spoon into egg white holes.

3. Serve and enjoy or refrigerate for future use.

Nutrition: Calories: 60 Protein: 3.1g Carbs: 1.8g Fat: 4.7g Saturated Fat: 1.1g Sodium: 34mg

21. **Tuna-Pasta Salad**

Preparation Time: 15 minutes

Cooking Time: 15 minutes

Servings: 4

Ingredients:

- 2 cups whole wheat macaroni, uncooked

- 2 5-oz cans low-sodium tuna, water pack - 1/3 cup diced onion

- ¼ cup sliced carrots

- ½ cup chopped zucchini

- ¼ cup fat free mayonnaise

- ¼ cup light sour cream

- ¼ tsp. pepper

Directions:

1. In a pot of boiling water, cook macaroni according to manufacturer's instructions minus the oil and salt.

2. Drain macaroni, run under cold tap water until cool and set aside.

3. Drain tuna and discard liquid.

4. Place tuna in a salad bowl.

5. Add zucchini, carrots, drained macaroni and onion. Toss to mix.

6. Add mayonnaise and sour cream. Mix well.

7. Season with pepper, serve and enjoy.

8. Serve and enjoy.

Nutrition: Calories: 174.4 Protein: 5.1g Carbs: 27.7g Fat: 4.8g Saturated Fat: 1.5gSodium: 54mg

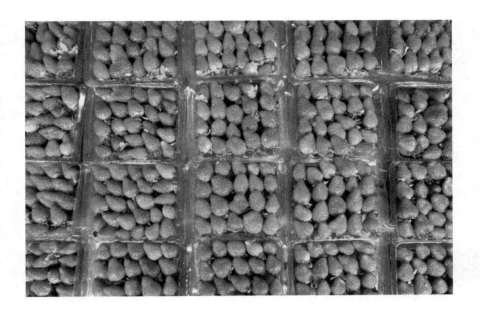

FISH & SEAFOOD

22. <u>Pressure Cooker "Low" Carb Manhattan Clam Chowder</u>

Preparation time: 25 minutes

Cooking time: 5 minutes

Servings: 4

Ingredients:

- 4 chopped strips of bacon

- 3 diced large carrots

- 3 diced stalks of celery

- 1 cleaned and diced red pepper

- 4 cloves of minced fresh garlic

- 1 tablespoon of dried oregano

- 1 teaspoon of Ground chili paste

- 1 and a ½ teaspoon of crushed sunflower seeds

- ¾ cup of fresh leeks diced

- 6 ounce of turnip peeled up and diced

- 10 trimmed and quartered radishes

- 16 ounce of clam juiced

- 28 ounce of diced tomatoes

- 15 ounce of crushed tomatoes

- 1 and a /12 tablespoon of tomato paste

- 2 pieces of bay leaves

- 3 can of 6 ounce chopped clams

- 3 tablespoon of fresh chopped parsley

- Crushed sunflower seeds

Directions:

1. Dice and cut up the veggies

2. Add carrots, celery, red pepper in a bowl and add leeks, radish and turnips to another bowl

3. Drain and separate the clams from clam juice and place the clams in fridge for later use

4. Make sure to reserve the clam juice

5. Set your pot to Sauté mode and add chopped bacon

6. Spread it evenly and leave for a few minutes

7. Once the bacon fat has turned brown, scrap off the browned bit and leave 2 tablespoon in the pot

8. Add leeks, sunflower seeds, pepper, carrots to the pot and Sauté for about 5 minutes

9. Add minced garlic, chili paste, sunflower seeds, thyme and oregano

10. Sauté for 1 minute more

11. Pour reserved Clam juice and both bottles of Clam juice, crushed tomato, tomato paste and diced tomatoes

12. Add radishes, bay leaves and turnips

13. Lock up the lid and cook on HIGH pressure for 5 minutes

14. Release the pressure naturally over 10 minutes

15. Remove the lid and stir in parsley and clam

16. Serve with a sprinkle of grated parmesan cheese

Nutrition: Calories: 730 Fat: 26g Carbohydrates: 58g Protein: 68g

23. **Spicy Pineapple Shrimp**

Preparation time: 10 minutes

Cooking time: 5 minutes

Servings: 4

Ingredients:

- 1 large sized red bell pepper, cleaned and sliced
- 12 ounce of Quinoa
- ½ a cup of unsweetened pineapple juice
- ¼ cup of dry white wine
- 2 tablespoon of soy sauce
- 2 tablespoon of Thai sweet chili sauce
- 1 pound of large shrimp
- 1 tablespoon of ground chili paste
- 4 chopped up scallions
- 1 and a ½ cups of unsweetened pineapple chunks

Directions:

1. Drain the juice from pineapple and set the pineapple chunks on the side
2. Measure out ½ a cup of pineapple juice

3. Add red bell pepper, pineapple juice, rice, wine, chili sauce, soy sauce, chili paste and chopped scallions to the Instant Pot

4. Place the shrimp on top

5. Lock up the lid and cook on HIGH pressure for 2 minutes

6. Naturally release the pressure over 10 minutes

7. Add pineapple chunks and scallion greens

8. Mix well and serve!

Nutrition: Calories: 299 Fat: 5g Carbohydrates: 54g Protein: 8g

24. **<u>Salmon and Broccoli Medley</u>**

Preparation time: 1 minute

Cooking time: 4 minutes

Servings: 4

Ingredients:

- 2 and a ½ ounce of Salmon fillet

- 2 and a ½ ounce of broccoli

- 9 ounce of new potatoes

- 1 teaspoon of butter

- Pepper as needed

- Crushed sunflower seeds

- Fresh herbs

Directions:

1. Chop the broccoli into florets and keep them on the side

2. ½ a cup of water to your Instant Pot

3. Season the potatoes with sunflower seeds, fresh herbs and pepper

4. Season the salmon and broccoli with sunflower seeds and pepper

5. Add potatoes to a steaming rack and smother them with butter

6. Transfer to your Instant Pot

7. Lock up the lid and cook for 2 minutes on the Steam setting

8. Quick release the pressure

9. Add broccoli florets and salmon and steam cook for 2 minutes more

10. Quick release

11. Serve and enjoy!

Nutrition: Calories: 701 Fat: 39g Carbohydrates: 30g Protein: 57g

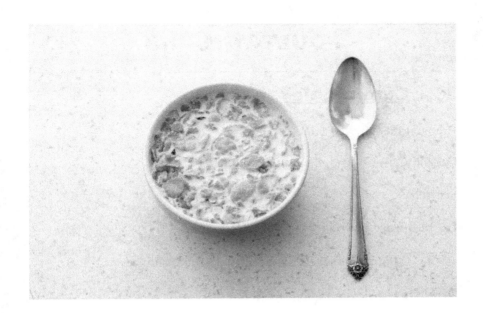

POULTRY MAINS

25. **Cumin Chicken**

Preparation time: 10 minutes

Cooking time: 1 hour

Servings: 6

Ingredients:

- 2 pounds chicken thighs, boneless and skinless

- 1 yellow onion, chopped

- 2 tablespoons olive oil

- 3 garlic cloves, minced

- 1 tablespoon coriander seeds, ground

- 1 teaspoon cumin, ground

- 1 cup low-sodium chicken stock

- 4 tablespoons chipotle chili paste

- A pinch of black pepper

- 1 tablespoon coriander, chopped

Directions:

1. Heat up a pan with the oil over medium heat; add the onion and the garlic and sauté for 5 minutes.

2. Add the meat and brown for 5 minutes more.

3. Add the rest of the ingredients, toss, introduce everything in the oven and bake at 390 degrees F for 50 minutes.

4. Divide the whole mix between plates and serve.

Nutrition: 372 calories, 44.9g protein, 6.4g carbohydrates, 17.6g fat, 0.5g fiber, 138mg cholesterol, 274mg sodium, 407mg potassium

26. **<u>Chives Chicken</u>**

Preparation time: 10 minutes

Cooking time: 25 minutes

Servings: 4

Ingredients:

- 2 chicken breasts, skinless, boneless and roughly cubed

- 3 red onions, sliced

- 2 tablespoons olive oil

- 1 cup low-sodium vegetable stock

- A pinch of black pepper

- 1 tablespoon cilantro, chopped

- 1 tablespoon chives, chopped

Directions:

1. Heat up a pan with the oil over medium heat; add the onions and a pinch of black pepper, and sauté for 10 minutes stirring often. Add the chicken and cook for 3 minutes more.

2. Add the rest of the ingredients, bring to a simmer and cook over medium heat for 12 minutes more.

3. Divide the chicken and onions mix between plates and serve.

Nutrition: 99 calories, 1.3g protein, 8.8g carbohydrates, 7.1g fat, 2.1g fiber, 0mg cholesterol, 39mg sodium, 158mg potassium

27. **<u>Turkey with Pepper and Rice</u>**

Preparation time: 10 minutes

Cooking time: 42 minutes

Servings: 4

Ingredients:

- 1 turkey breast, skinless, boneless and cubed

- 1 cup white rice

- 2 cups low-sodium vegetable stock

- 1 teaspoon hot paprika

- 2 small Serrano peppers, chopped

- 2 garlic cloves, minced

- 2 tablespoons olive oil

- ½ red bell pepper chopped

- A pinch of black pepper

Directions: Heat up a pan with the oil over medium heat; add the Serrano peppers and garlic and sauté for 2 minutes. Add the meat and brown it for 5 minutes. Add the rice and the other ingredients bring to a simmer and cook over medium heat for 35 minutes. Stir, divide between plates and serve.

Nutrition: 245 calories, 4g protein, 40.2g carbohydrates, 7.3g fat, 1.3g fiber, 0mg cholesterol, 76mg sodium, 134mg potassium

BEEF AND PORK MAINS

28. **Beef Brisket**

Preparation Time: 15 minutes

Cooking Time: 8 hours

Servings: About 12

Ingredients:

- 5 pounds Beef Brisket (trimmed)

- 2 minced cloves Garlic

- ½ tsp. Black Pepper

- 2 tbsp. Brown Sugar

- 2 tsp. Paprika (smoked)

- 2 sliced Onions

- 1 ½ cup Beef Broth

- 3 diced Carrots

- 3 sliced Parsnips

- 14 ounces diced Tomatoes

Directions:

1. In a bowl, mix paprika, brown sugar, black pepper and garlic.

2. Coat beef with paprika mixture and place it into the slow cooker.

3. Now, place all the remaining Ingredients in layers.

4. Cook on "low" for 8 hours.

5. Transfer the beef to a cutting board.

6. Leave it for 10 minutes at least.

7. Slice and serve with the cooked vegetables.

Nutrition: 283 Calories 15 g Total Fat 128 mg Cholesterol 385 mg Sodium 7 mg Carbohydrates 2 g Dietary Fiber 44 g Protein

29. **Lemony Pork Roast**

Preparation Time: 15 minutes

Cooking Time: 8 hours 15 minutes

Servings: About 8

Ingredients:

- 4 boneless Pork Chops

- Ground Black Pepper

- 1 sliced Onion

- 2 tsp. Olive Oil

- 1 minced clove Garlic

- 1 sliced Red Bell Pepper

- ½ tsp. ground Cumin

- ½ tsp. ground Cinnamon

- ½ cup Chicken Broth

- ½ cup Coconut Milk

- 1 diced tart Apple

- 1 cup cubed Squash

- 2 tbsp. chopped Parsley

Directions:

1. Place all Ingredients except Pork Chops in the slow cooker.

2. Put the pork chops in afterwards.

3. Cook on "low" for 8 hours.

4. When cooked, transfer the pork to a cutting board.

5. Leave it for 10 minutes and then slice.

6. Transfer the pork and vegetables to heated plates and serve.

Nutrition: 317 Calories 15 g Total Fat 106 mg Cholesterol 174 mg Sodium 12 mg Carbohydrates 5 g Dietary Fiber 49 g Protein

SNACKS

30. **Dill Zucchini Spread**

Preparation time: 5 minutes

Cooking time: 10 minutes

Servings: 4

Ingredients:

- ½ cup nonfat yogurt

- 2 zucchinis, chopped

- 1 tablespoon olive oil

- 2 spring onions, chopped

- ¼ cup low-sodium vegetable stock

- 2 garlic cloves, minced

- 1 tablespoon dill, chopped

- A pinch of nutmeg, ground

Directions:

1. Heat up a pan with the oil over medium heat; add the onions and garlic, stir and sauté for 3 minutes.

2. Add the zucchinis and the other ingredients except the yogurt, toss, cook for 7 minutes more and take off the heat.

3. Add the yogurt, blend using an immersion blender, divide into bowls and serve.

Nutrition: 75 calories, 3.4g protein, 7.2g carbohydrates, 4.1g fat, 1.5g fiber, 2mg cholesterol, 43mg sodium, 389mg potassium

31. **Seeds Bowls**

Preparation time: 10 minutes

Cooking time: 20 minutes

Servings: 4

Ingredients:

- 2 tablespoons olive oil
- 1 teaspoon smoked paprika
- 1 cup sunflower seeds
- 1 cup chia seeds
- 2 apples, cored and cut into wedges
- ½ teaspoon cumin, ground
- A pinch of cayenne pepper

Directions:

1. In a bowl, combine the seeds with the apples and the other ingredients, toss, spread on a lined baking sheet, introduce in the oven and bake at 350 degrees F for 20 minutes.

2. Divide into bowls and serve as a snack.

Nutrition: 291 calories, 6.3g protein, 27.1g carbohydrates, 19.8g fat, 11.2g fiber, 0mg cholesterol, 6mg sodium, 297mg potassium

32. **Tahini Pumpkin Dip**

Preparation time: 5 minutes

Cooking time: 0 minutes

Servings: 4

Ingredients:

- 2 cups pumpkin flesh

- ½ cup pumpkin seeds

- 1 tablespoon lemon juice

- 1 tablespoon sesame seed paste

- 1 tablespoon olive oil

Directions:

1. In a blender, combine the pumpkin with the seeds and the other ingredients, pulse well, divide into bowls and serve a party spread.

Nutrition: 162 calories, 5.5g protein, 9.7g carbohydrates, 12.7g fat, 2.3g fiber, 0mg cholesterol, 5mg sodium, 436mg potassium

DESSERTS

33. **Tart Raspberry Crumble Bar**

Preparation Time: 50 minutes

Cooking Time: 45 minutes

Servings: 9

Ingredients:

- 1/2 cup whole toasted almonds

- 1 3/4 cups whole wheat flour

- 1/4 teaspoon salt

- 3/4 cup cold, unsalted butter, cut into cubes

- 3 tablespoons cold water, or more if needed

- 1/2 cup granulated sugar

- 18-ounce fresh raspberries

Directions:

1. In a food processor, pulse almonds until chopped coarsely. Transfer to a bowl.

2. Add flour and salt into food processor and pulse until a bit combined. Add butter and pulse until you have a coarse batter. Evenly divide batter into two bowls.

3. In first bowl of batter, knead well until it forms a ball. Wrap in cling wrap, flatten a bit and chill for an hour for easy handling.

4. In second bowl of batter, add sugar. In a pinching motion, pinch batter to form clusters of streusel. Set aside.

5. When ready to bake, preheat oven to 375oF and lightly grease an 8x8-inch baking pan with cooking spray.

6. Discard cling wrap and evenly press dough on bottom of pan, up to 1-inch up the sides of the pan, making sure that everything is covered in dough.

7. Evenly spread raspberries. Top with streusel.

8. Pop in the oven and bake until golden brown and berries are bubbly, around 45 minutes.

9. Remove from oven and cool for 20 minutes before slicing into 9 equal bars.

10. Serve and enjoy or store in a lidded container for 10-days in the fridge.

Nutrition: Calories: 235.7 Protein: 4.4g Carbs: 29.1g Fat: 11.3g Saturated Fat: 6.5g Sodium: 73mg

34. **Easy Coconut-Carrot Cake Balls**

Preparation Time: 10 minutes

Cooking Time: 0 minutes

Servings: 16

Ingredients:

- 3/4 cup peeled and finely shredded carrot

- 1 cup packed pitted medjool dates

- 1 ¾ cups raw walnuts

- 3/4 tsp. ground cinnamon

- 1/2 tsp. ground ginger

- 1 pinch ground nutmeg

- 2 tsp. vanilla extract

- 5 tbsp. almond flour

- 1/4 cup raisins

- ¼ cup desiccated coconut flakes

Directions:

1. In food processor, process dates until it clumps. Transfer to a bowl.

2. In same food processor, process walnuts, cinnamon, ginger, and nutmeg. Process until it resembles a fine meal.

3. Add the processed dates, extract, almond flour, and shredded carrots. Pulse until you form a loose dough but not mushy. Do not over-pulse. Transfer to a bowl.

4. Pulse desiccated coconut into tinier flakes and transfer to a small plate.

5. Divide the carrot batter into 4 and then divide each part into 4 to make a total of 16 equal sized balls.

6. Roll the balls in the coconut flakes, place in a lidded contained, and refrigerate for 2 hours before enjoying.

7. Can be stored in the fridge for a week and up to a month in the freezer.

Nutrition: Calories: 77.9 Protein: 1.5g Carbs: 3.8g Fat: 6.3g Saturated Fat: 1g Sodium: 8mg

CHRISTMAS & EASTER RECIPES

35. **Sweet Avocado Bowl**

Preparation time: 6 minutes

Cooking time: 1 hour

Servings: 2

Ingredients:

- 2 cups avocado, peeled, pitted and cubed
- 1 cup coconut cream
- 1 tablespoon maple syrup
- 12 figs, halved
- ½ cup almonds, chopped
- 1 teaspoon vanilla extract

Directions:

1. In your slow cooker, mix the avocado with the cream, maple syrup and the other ingredients, put the lid on, cook on High for 1 hour, divide into bowls and serve.

Nutrition: Calories 1027, Fat 70g, Cholesterol 0mg, Sodium 40mg, Carbohydrate 104.1g, Fiber 26.6g, Sugars 66.6g, Protein 14.3g, Potassium 1997mg

36. **<u>Brown Cake</u>**

Preparation time: 10 minutes

Cooking time: 2 hours and 30 minutes

Servings: 8

Ingredients:

- 1 cup flour

- 1 and ½ cup stevia

- ½ cup chocolate almond milk

- 2 teaspoons baking powder

- 1 and ½ cups hot water

- ¼ cup cocoa powder+ 2 tablespoons

- 2 tablespoons canola oil

- 1 teaspoon vanilla extract

- Cooking spray

Directions:

1. In a bowl, mix flour with ¼-cup cocoa, baking powder, almond milk, oil and vanilla extract, whisk well and spread on the bottom of the slow cooker greased with cooking spray.

2. In a separate bowl, mix stevia with the water and the rest of the cocoa, whisk well, spread over the batter, cover, and cook your cake on High for 2 hours and 30 minutes.

3. Leave the cake to cool down, slice and serve.

Nutrition: Calories 150, Fat 7.6g, Cholesterol 1mg, Sodium 7mg, Carbohydrate 56.8g, Fiber 1.8g, Sugars 4.4g, Protein 2.9g, Potassium 185mg

37. **Soft Pudding**

Preparation time: 6 minutes

Cooking time: 1 hour

Servings: 4

Ingredients:

- ½ cup coconut water

- 2 teaspoons lime zest, grated

- 2 tablespoons green tea powder

- 1 and ½ cup avocado, pitted, peeled and chopped

- 1 tablespoon stevia

Directions:

1. In your slow cooker, mix coconut water with avocado, green tea powder, lime zest and stevia, stir, cover, cook on Low for 1 hour, divide into bowls and serve.

Nutrition: Calories 120, Fat 10.7g, Cholesterol 0mg, Sodium 35mg, Carbohydrate 8.5g, Fiber 4.4g, Sugars 1.1g, Protein 1.5g, Potassium 362mg

THANKSGIVING RECIPES

38. **Crusted Salmon**

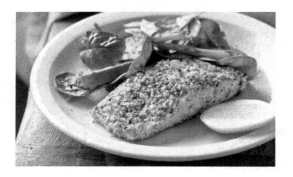

Preparation time: 5 minutes

Cooking time: 15 minutes

Servings: 6

Ingredients:

- 6 salmon fillets;

- 1 garlic clove, minced;

- 1/3 cup sour cream;

- 2/3 cup dry breadcrumbs;

- 2/3 cup pistachios, chopped;

- 1/2 cup shallots, minced;

- 2 tablespoons olive oil;

- 2 tablespoons horseradish;

- 1 tablespoon fresh dill, chopped;

- 1/2 teaspoon lemon zest;

- 1/4 teaspoon crushed red pepper flakes.

Directions:

1. Preheat the oven to 350 °F. Prepare a baking pan and coat with cooking spray.
2. Place the salmon into the pan skin side down.
3. Mix garlic, breadcrumbs, pistachios, shallots, olive oil, horseradish, dill, lemon zest, and red pepper flakes in a bowl.
4. Top each salmon fillet with sour cream and breadcrumbs mixture.
5. Bake for 13-15 minutes and serve.

Nutrition: 376 calories; 25.2 g fat; 15.1 g carbohydrate; 24.3 g protein; 219 mg sodium; 2.0 g fiber.

39.   **Creamy Pasta with Shrimp**

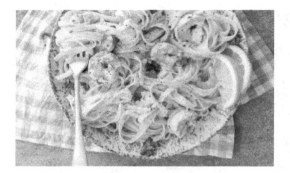

Preparation time: 20 minutes

Cooking time: 20 minutes

Servings: 4

Ingredients:

- 8 oz. whole-wheat fettuccine pasta;

- 12 oz. shrimp, peeled and deveined;

- 4 cups arugula;

- 1 tablespoon extra-virgin olive oil;

- 2 tablespoons butter, unsalted;

- 1 tablespoon garlic, chopped;

- 1/4 teaspoon crushed red pepper;

- 1/4 cup low-fat plain yogurt;

- 1 teaspoon lemon zest;

- 2 tablespoons lemon juice;

- 1/3 cup Parmesan cheese, grated;

- 1/4 cup fresh basil, sliced.

Directions:

1. Bring a saucepan of water to a boil and add pasta. Cook until al dente and drain.

2. Preheat olive oil in a pan over medium heat. Add shrimp and cook for about 2-3 minutes. Remove from the pan.

3. Melt butter in the same pan and add garlic and red pepper, cook for about 1 minute. Add arugula and cook for 1 minute more.

4. Add pasta, yogurt, and lemon zest, add water if pasta is too thick. Toss well to coat and add shrimp and lemon juice. Serve topped with basil and cheese.

Nutrition: 403 calories; 14.4 g fat; 46.2 g carbohydrate; 28.1 g protein; 396 mg sodium; 6.1 g fiber.

40. **Fish Tacos**

Preparation time: 10 minutes

Cooking time: 20 minutes Servings: 6

Ingredients:

- 12 corn tortillas;

- 6 white fish fillets (6 oz.);

- 2 cups red cabbage, chopped;

- 1 cup fresh cilantro, chopped;

- 1/4 cup olive oil;

- 1 teaspoon ground cardamom;

- 1 teaspoon paprika;

- 1 teaspoon pepper;

- 2 limes cut into wedges.

Directions:

1. Preheat oven to 400 °F. Coat a baking dish with cooking spray.Mix olive oil, cardamom, paprika, and pepper in a bowl. Add fish and toss well to coat, marinate for 30 minutes. Transfer fish to the baking dish and cook for 15-20 minutes. Divide the fish fillets among tortillas, top with cabbage, cilantro, and lime juice. Serve.

Nutrition: 284 calories; 5.1 g fat; 26.2 g carbohydrate; 35.4 g protein; 278 mg sodium; 4.2 g fiber.

CONCLUSION

Thank you for making it to the end. Living with hypertension can be a stressful challenge as it is associated with several other life-threatening diseases and health problems such as heart diseases, diabetes and renal diseases. Hypertension is also referred as silent killer. But diet and lifestyle changes can have a major impact on managing these issues. DASH diet is designed with two different levels of sodium. The first level for reducing sodium in diet was 2300 mg per day and the second level was 1500 mg which was the ultimate target to cut down on sodium content. Prehypertension can be controlled by the diet and physical activity alone.

Medication is only suggested to those who are at higher risk of getting a stroke or any other associated complication. Individuals who are overweight or obese are at higher risk of being affected by these health issues. Exercise and dietary modifications can help in reducing the weight and controlling the blood pressure. Keeping track of your performance in relation to exercise or physical activity can help you keep motivated for a longer period of time. Similarly, dietary record is also helpful in estimating the daily intake and calories consumed per day.

Excluding the habits of using salt shaker and avoiding high sodium packaged products can help sodium intake in moderation. Diet as suggested by the dietary approaches to stop hypertension (DASH) is low in sodium, fat and sugar content and high in fiber, protein and fresh and organic food products that ultimately help to improve the overall health of a person. Weight reduction has been proven to reduce the occurrence of other diseases that are associated with high blood pressure, for example it will prevent the premature stiffening of the arteries and will reduce the risk of stroke or heart attack.

The DASH strategy is a new way to eat — for a living. When you slip a few days off the eating plan, don't let it keep you from reaching your health goals.

Ask yourself why you got off-track.

Get on track again. Here's how: Tell yourself why you've gone off track. Was it drinking at a party? Have you experienced tension at home, or at work? Find out what started your side track and then begin the DASH plan again.

Look out for if you tried to do too much at once.

Anyone starting a new lifestyle sometimes tries to change too much at once. Instead, one or two things should be changed at a time. The only way to succeed is, slowly but surely.

Break down the process to small steps.

Not only does this discourage you from having to do too much at once but it also makes the changes easier. Break complicated objectives into smaller, easier measures, each achievable.

Write it down.

Keep record of what you eat and what you do. That can help you figure out the issue. Keep record for a few days. For example, you may find that you eat high-fat foods while watching TV. If so, you might start eating a substitute snack instead of the high-fat foods on hand. The record also allows you to be sure that each food group and every day physical activity is being enough.

Feast for performance.

For your accomplishments, treat yourself to a non-food treat.

Losing weight

DASH can easily be adapted to a weight loss plan as it contains tons of fiber content, is protein-balanced, restricts waste, and is relatively low in fat.

DASH's concept is that the food you eat can be as simplistic or as complicated as you wish. It is convenient for just about anyone, and although it has not been developed or tested for vegetarians or those with milk allergy, it can easily be modified to suit your needs.

CPSIA information can be obtained
at www.ICGtesting.com
Printed in the USA
BVHW091717250521
608095BV00004B/1058